I Secretly

WANTED TO DIE

I Secretly
WANTED TO DIE

A (completely) Different Story about C A N C E R

Saskia Mevis and her Miraculous Body

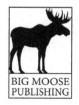

BIG MOOSE
PUBLISHING

This Book is dedicated to those who are wondering,
"What else is possible?"

For all the Bodies who are living on this Planet, have ever lived on this Planet
and will be living on this Planet...

For the Bodies that have not only sustained us, but also inspired us, and even
tolerated our stupidity and our hard-headedness against everything that
they know is possible about life and living, that we kept refusing lifetime after
lifetime.

And specifically, to my wonderful Body, for inviting me to step up and step into
so much more living; for having my back, and for speaking through me in name
of all bodies to create this Book in front of you.

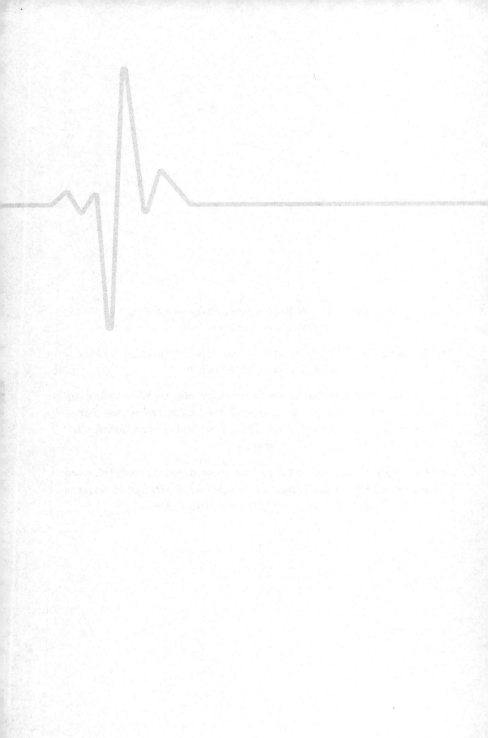

Contents

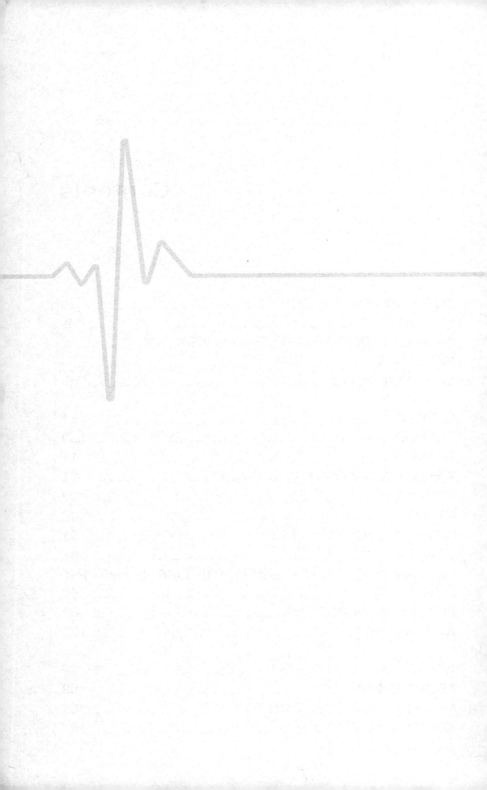

Acknowledgments

I am beyond words, indescribably grateful for all my personal angels with and without bodies that accompanied me on this exploration of consciousness and always, no matter what it looks like or what I have decided about it, have my back!

I am humbly grateful for my Body, for having my back even when I was not having its...and inviting and inspiring me to keep going in the direction of more Greatness, more Possibilities, more LIVING!

To each and every person that crossed my path in this adventure, you have contributed in your own unique way. A smile from a stranger, a judgment from a doctor, a conversation with a friend or anything in between has contributed to what I am willing to be and know today.

"Everything that ends with more awareness ends well."
– Dr. Dain Heer

And last, but not least, my infinite gratitude for this body of work called Access Consciousness® and in particular Dr. Dain Heer, Gary Douglas, and Shannon O'Hara in cooperation with Talk To The Entities®. Without them having my back and being willing to pioneer towards spaces and places that are resisted and rejected the most, just because they KNEW there must be something else available for living on this planet, I can safely say, I would have killed my Body...

GRATEFUL...

Foreword

by Gabi van Putten

Is there something whispering in you that knows that more is possible?

We can ignore these whispers for a long time, but eventually they will find a way out. The point is that we often see this as something negative at first, because it doesn't always present itself in the nicest way. Sometimes those whispers turn into screams...even disease.

I know that very well... by the time I was 31, I had 10 diagnoses added to my name. I was like, "OK, this is enough!"

I've been collecting diagnoses for 13 years now and I'm done, even though I've always dealt with them differently. I was always looking for the possibilities with my Body and just knew that all these diagnoses were not congruent with who I was. Still, there was a common thread where I started seeing diagnoses as an invitation to look for more of me...although I didn't see it that way at first.

Looking for more of me through my diagnoses was not the easiest way and involved a lot of judgment and suffering. I was done with that in 2018 and I only now realize that I made the demand I was going to do things differently with my Body. No more labels and diagnoses as an excuse to be more of me anymore. I chose to explore who I can truly be from the perspective of possibilities and not from limitations and fixing myself.

I still learn every day and I realize that communicating with my Body is perhaps the greatest adventure of embodiment! There are days that I don't even know what to do with my Body and all the intensity that is there... there are days when I soften and melt with my Body. It all started when I refused to see myself and my Body as a victim of life any longer.

It is wonderful to see and hear how we all have our own adventure with our bodies and I would very much like to invite you to such a special exploration...

In this beautiful book, Saskia takes us to the Possibilities beyond the Impossible!

I have had the honor to work with her for almost 2 years now and she has inspired me to create something else with my Body. This woman is a powerhouse and, at the same time, so kind. She embodies a space where you cannot go to the wrongness of you anymore. Her 'cancer adventure' invited her only more and more to explore her amazing capacities with bodies and possibilities.

This book is a gift to everybody, and you and your Body are warmly invited to receive exactly that what will create a greater life for you. Enjoy!

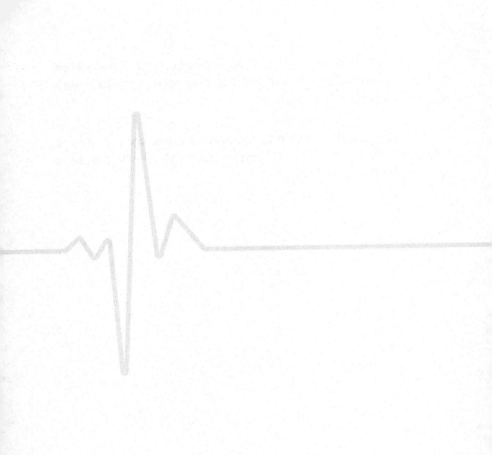

A Note to the Reader

Throughout this book you will see the word "body" capitalized. This is done intentionally to acknowledge the miraculous entity that walks through life with us as having its own consciousness, gifts, and capacities.

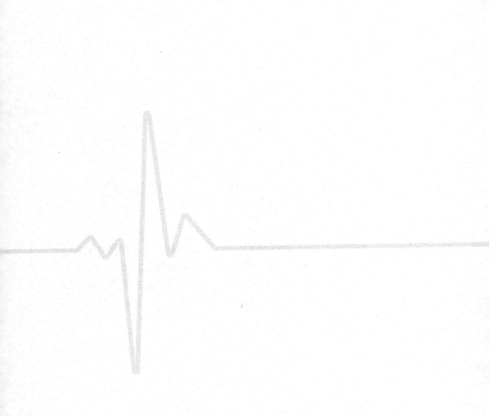

An *Invitation* to a
Different Possibility

What you are about to read might seem to be the weirdest, most off the planet, insane thing you have come across until now, or is it?

FOR WHOM AM I WRITING THIS? YOU!

There is a reason why you have been drawn to read this. It might have been waiting for you! You might have been asking for this in one way or another.

Whether you have dealt with or are dealing with cancer in your Body or anybody you hold very dear who is dealing with it... Whether you are suffering or someone you care about is

suffering any kind of disease...
Or you just desire to have a different perspective on what seems to be the most terrible thing that could ever happen to you...

The information in this book might give you a different perspective and moreover a different Possibility.

I purposely write "that could ever happen to you" because this is one of the greatest lies that keeps you from creating a life that is truly worth living, and from changing anything that does not work for you.

Nothing ever happens to you...it is a set of choices that you made consciously and mostly unconsciously based on your own points of view or ones that you took on from other people.

YOU CAN ALWAYS MAKE A DIFFERENT CHOICE.

I would like to invite you to something that is different... something that will empower you beyond anything that you ever seen, and you always secretly deep down knew to be true!
I would love for you to know that everything you learn about your Body and diseases is based on concluding disasters, which keeps you from knowing that YOU, yes YOU, can change everything that you desire to change.

If you desperately need to hold on to the fact that you are a victim of what happened to you, you might really dislike me after reading this, or maybe you might not even read on! Yet...

WHAT IF THERE IS ANOTHER POSSIBILITY?

Prologue

If you would have told me a few years ago, "You are going to write a book!" I would have said, "You are crazy!"
First, I am totally dyslexic.
Second, I do not have the capacity to write.
And third, no, I just cannot do that.

In fact, this book has been knocking on my door for over two years and every time we tried to create it, it just didn't happen.
What do I mean by 'we'?
My Body and I wrote this book, together, and even acknowledging this makes my Body giggle. My Body is like; "Of course I am writing this book with you."

Have you ever really acknowledged that you have a possibility for co-creation and cooperation with your Body? For me, it's something new that I have started to acknowledge more and more.

What if today it's about what you know and what your Body knows? What do you know together?

Once I acknowledged I wasn't alone in writing this book, everything changed and I just started. Looking at what it has become and what we created based on what I know, what my Body knows and what the book wanted to be, I am in such gratitude and awe.

I also must acknowledge that this is not only a book. It might look like a book, it might show up like a book, but it's also something else. I sensed every molecule in my Universe changing with what we put on paper.

I hope that this book will be a bridge from the unconscious to the Conscious World. When I tap into the energy of the Book, it's this little joyful Beast for everybody who's looking for it. This book will find people, as it found you... and it will be found.

NOW IS THE TIME AND NOW IS THE SPACE!

Introduction

This is the story of how I became acquainted with the Universe having my back and creating something different with cancer and my Body.

I was at the airport, onwards to a different possibility, when this song started playing.

I'm allowing
Me to be me
I'm allowing
Me to be free
I'm allowing my power
I'm allowing well being
I'm allowing my path to light up before me

I'm allowing, everything to just be as it comes to me
I'm shining brightly
I'm allowing, easily allowing all my dreams to be
In the right timing
I'm allowing my worth
I'm allowing my brilliance
I'm allowing my path
To unfold now before me
I'm allowing, everything to just be as it comes to me
I'm shining brightly
I'm allowing, easily allowing all my dreams to be
In the right timing
- Alexia Chellun[1]

It was at that moment the Universe showered me with: "Hey, I got you!"

This is one of the greatest gifts that I got to receive over the last few years...

That the Universe truly has our back if we allow it.

Many of us just see it as a nice concept, while believing that it is not so.

One of the demands I made for me, and I would like to invite you to...

WHAT WOULD IT TAKE TO TRULY KNOW THE UNIVERSE HAS MY BACK?

[1] Allowing, by Alexia Chellun, from the album *Just Before I Sleep*, (P)&(C)2018

YOUR BODY KNOWS...WHEN YOU START LIVING YOUR TRUTH, YOUR BODY WILL BE HEALING BEYOND ANYTHING EVER SEEN BEFORE, EVEN IF THAT MEANS DYING!

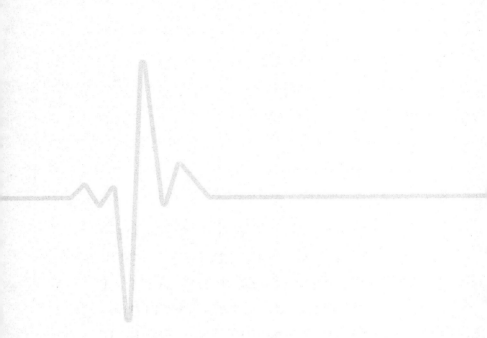

Cancer

I secretly wanted to die...

"I was scared out of my mind
It was really hard
I made the decision to not give into the fear
I chose to keep living!"
- The Flash

I would very much like to invite you to a special exploration that started for me in October 2019.

"Miss Mevis, you have Thyroid Cancer and if you will not let us operate on you, you will die..."

My life stood still for a good few weeks, like one big error that seemed to be unreal...Walking out of the hospital screaming, "F*ck!" for about 50 times...people might have thought I went insane. ☺

Truth be told, I thought I had gone insane.

Cancer...CANCER...CAAAANNCERRRR...

Even the word brings your world into an error...

It goes hand in hand with Death, Dying, and Suffering.

Often it happens to other people... most of us even had it happen to people we care about a lot...

But now it was different. It happened to me...and it might have happened to you.

Do you notice how the word "happens" kind of keeps jumping at you?

It is because that is one of the programs that is extremely difficult to go beyond, if you don't have the information that I am about to expose to you in this book.

This world tells you Magic is not real...

It will tell you that you need to protect yourself against dying...

It will make you believe that horrible things can happen to you!

That we are subject to what happens to us and, in this case, our bodies.

We are told disease happens to you, and you are the victim of it...

It needs to go away; you need to fight it; you need to fix it; you need it to be different.

All the while secretly functioning from the point of view that you don't really have a say in this. That you would have to be very lucky to change or survive this horrible thing that happened to you and, let's be honest, how many of us believe that we would be that special?

DO YOU VALUE YOU? DO YOU KNOW YOU ARE SPECIAL?

I have had a little lump in my neck for years. It never really worried me, until one moment when I walked out of my yoga school after an evening of teaching, and I got a clear sense to go see a doctor now.

This process by itself was already very fascinating because the first doctor I saw said, "No, it's nothing."
The second one said, "Oh, let's do a test."
The third was like, "No, I don't think it's anything."
Then the fourth one literally sat me down and said, "I have a very bad diagnosis for you.
It's Thyroid Cancer."

At that moment it was like someone banged my head against the wall and the only thing that I remember was like, fuck, fuck, fuck, fighting to stay present and not faint.
I walked out of that hospital like a Gilles de la Tourette Person with tears pouring down my face.

Here is another universal law. You are psychic and whether you know it or not you are also very capable of perceiving other people's thoughts, feelings, and emotions. You are like one big psychic SpongeBob being able to perceive A LOT, ALL THE TIME!

Within a nanosecond, I downloaded all the drama, all the suffering, all the intensity of everybody who had cancer, dealt with cancer and is dealing with cancer, past present and future. I stuck myself in the box of impossibilities and it was like I couldn't move anymore.

It took a few days of intense suffering.
To be quite honest with you, I didn't know which way was up anymore. Here is this professional doctor saying that if I will not receive the operation, I will for sure die and still there is nothing in my world that makes me want to choose this operation. My Body was so clear from moment number one that we were not doing this operation. I just couldn't. There was massive pressure from the doctors and this reality for me to do whatever they decided was right for me.

I remember asking my doctor, "How many people just get the operation because you tell them it is a good idea?" He looked puzzled at me, and answered: "Everybody."
And the weird thing was, I just could not go ahead with it... I just could not.
You know how sometimes you wish you could do something and there is just no way in your Universe that you can?

This was what was going on for me.
Having my throat be cut open 10 inches (25 cm), having my thyroid and 15 lymph nodes taken out, needing to go into radioactive quarantine and having to take hormones for the rest of my life just did not match with what I knew about diseases. It did not match with what I knew about me!

I had been diagnosed with chronic not changeable diseases before, that I did change. They weren't cancer, but they were definitely incurable according to the professionals.

Let me make a little side note here!
I respect doctors and I honor their knowledge. Nothing of

what I am about to write makes them wrong or less valuable. I believe we can be extremely grateful for modern medicine, and it can be a great contribution to our Bodies and the quality of life and living, when used from that space of contribution. If you are bleeding to death because you lost a limb, GO TO THE HOSPITAL ☺ !

What I learned over the years in my own experience is that many times, unfortunately, it has not been seen as a gift of contribution, but a source for saving, which means we do not have to truly look at what is going on for us and our Bodies... which means we don't have to look at what is truly underneath that horrible thing that supposedly happened to us.

We choose to make doctors, specialists, professionals, and surgeons the source of fixing while making ourselves completely subject to their points of view and their way of looking at the world. We make them greater and bigger than ourselves, and more over, we decide they know more than us. After all, they studied and you did not.

Just for the record, this is another program we are functioning from: Everybody knows more than you do, which makes you always look outside of you for the answers. It will make sure you always will reach outside of you to make the right choice! Trying to make the right choice based on information from sources outside of you, to make sure you are not making the wrong choice, is another nicely imbedded program which will make you loop into oblivion.
Any of this sound familiar?

Let me tell you this. Nobody knows more about what is going on for you and your Body than you!

I had to start asking what was true for me. So in this case, my invitation to you is, "What do you know?"

YOU ARE THE ONLY PROFESSIONAL WHEN IT COMES TO YOU AND YOUR BODY! YOU KNOW!

Back to my "Fuck Fuck Fuck" state of going insane. That went on for a few days, then the light switched on. I just knew from the core of my being this could not be it...and here is where my journey started down the road of knowing that there MUST be another possibility...

So here was the choice presented to me.
I was going to buy into the fact that my disease was incurable without a very invasive operation. Which, for the record, they will make sound like it is nothing, yet it contracts your gut completely and makes you want to vomit. This, my friend, is a voice of your Body screaming at you, "DON'T GO THERE PLEASE!!!!"

We will talk more about this later in the book, but anything that will make your life and your future greater will have a sense of lightness and ease to it. May it be clear that this was not ease or light for me and my Body. Again, in your case, it might be a massive contribution to receive modern medicine treatment and if so, please go for it. Just know that what will create ease and greater for you always has a sense of lightness to it and you and your Body know!

The other choice was starting to look for what was true for me, even if nobody could see...

NOBODY KNOWS WHAT IS TRUE FOR YOU!

I started asking myself: What else is possible here and what do I know?

Was this always Easy? No, it most absolutely was not!

Yet did it GIFT me more awareness than I ever thought was possible?

Hell Yes!

I started exploring possibilities beyond the diagnosis, and now is the space and the time to get this energy into the world! Please receive my magnanimous gratitude for you and the fact that you picked up this book. No matter what you get out of it, I know it will for sure infuse a sense of greatness and a sense of possibilities in your world, if you are willing to receive it.

WHAT IS THIS BOOK LOOKING TO GIFT YOU? ARE YOU WILLING TO RECEIVE?

Choices

There I was diagnosed with thyroid cancer in desperate need for an immediate operation or I would die ...I didn't take the operation... and I am still alive as I am writing this... obviously! ☺

WHAT DO YOU KNOW?

Please don't take any of what you are reading here as the truth. Still, I am inviting you to get to what makes YOUR world lighter! What nobody teaches you is that you always, always, always (have I mentioned ALWAYS?) know what is real and true for you and that basically everything in this world is set up to make you believe that you don't.

This book is looking to create a different possibility, for you and your Body, for the World, and for this beautiful Planet.

What if there is a space in which you and only you always know what is real and true for you and you don't have to buy into anybody else's opinions or as they might call it...facts?

WHAT IF EVERYTHING THAT SHOWS UP IN YOUR WORLD IS BASED ON A CHOICE YOU MADE?

First, we will have to acknowledge one of the least popular laws of the Universe.
You might hate it too at first, but you will start loving it later, I promise.
The acknowledgement of choice!

Everything that shows up in your world is based on the points of view that you have.
Let me give you an easy example!
If you have the point of view that a certain disease can kill you... it will.
If you have the point of view that you can heal everything... you will.

So, the fact of the matter is that nobody can change your points of view for you.
The only thing they can do is invite you to look at yours and reconsider them...

Let's cut to the chase!
I created cancer in my Body.
And I know you might think, "What does she mean, created?"

It is exactly this that gave me the greatest key to turn my life around after being diagnosed.

We create diseases in our Body because of secret and hidden points of view. You know, the ones that you've buried deep down, because they are too ugly to look at.

So here is the ugly truth about cancer.

Someone that creates cancer is looking to die.

They have decided that their life is not worth living and that they don't have the capacity to turn it around and change it...

I was there...and I didn't want to look at it...
Until I was vulnerable enough to know...

I created cancer because I did not believe I could create a life worth living...I was stuck in a life that from the outside looked wondrous, beautiful, exciting, and definitely close to right! Let's face it, as a little side note, your most important task on this planet is to get your life right according to the perfect picture of what you have decided (and learned from your family) is right! Or...is it?

Which brings us to the title of this book: I Secretly Wanted to Die.

Not only secret to the outside world but also mostly secret to myself...

I forgot to give myself the memo: "Hey sweetie, I am choosing to die, as I don't believe my life is worth living or at the very least, that I can create it in a way that it is worth living!"

ARE YOU WILLING TO BE BRUTALLY HONEST WITH YOU?

Are you dying to get out of some stuck situation?
After I was willing to look at my own "ugly" truth more and

more I started seeing how most people live according to the principle of being "okay" without reaching for greatness.

Money, relationships, family, business and bodies are the most common things we settle and suffer in... because somewhere along the way we stopped reaching for more and started settling for less!

You know the concept... when you choose something, you have to stick with it!

PLEASE DON'T! You can choose again, all the time, and there is no choice, not even one, that you are not allowed to change. Even if everybody tries to tell you that you can't!

You my friend will never be "okay" with an "okay" life...as long you are not reaching for Greater, more Ease, more Joy, more Magic every single day, you are dying.

You are not meant to be mediocre, you are not meant to be okay.

YOU ARE MEANT TO BE GREAT!

What is Magic? People often dismiss it as something that is not real. It is something that shows up with glitter and unicorns, or maybe even only in fairytales. Let me introduce you to what I see as Magic.

Imagine...a place where everything is just wonderful... You are happy all the time, your Body is nurtured and you are enjoying every minute of your life...There is no judgment, no suffering, no limitations, no need and unbelievable but true... NO PROBLEMS. It is a place where you are carried by the magnanimous Universe and you explore a capacity to shift, change, create and generate everything you desire!

There is no right or wrong and people can be free from all

the trauma, drama and suffering. It's a space where there is a possibility for everyone to live with Ease, Joy and Glory.

You will find Magic in the big and little things around you and you are continuously invited to step into your greatness.

This is a place where receiving and gratitude are normal... where you can keep asking for more and keep upgrading your life!

It is place where life is worth living!

This is Magic to me...

YOU ARE MEANT FOR MAGIC!

It all starts with the acknowledgement of choice, because when you do, EVERYTHING can change. It is one of the most empowering gifts you can gift yourself.

For me this has been key, to keep on expanding my consciousness and let go of as many insane points of view as I possibly could.

For a long time, I had decided I could not say what I knew about disease.

I was not willing to offend people, or hurt people...or even lose people.

But what if we all have a unique knowing about what is possible and with you not saying it, you keep the world from having it?

WOULD YOU BE WILLING TO EMPOWER YOU BY THE ACKNOWLEDGEMENT OF CHOICE?

The acknowledgement of choice is one of the most empowering choices you can gift yourself!

Now here is an important side note. You cannot force this information on anybody that is not willing to receive it or looking for this information. Just because you have decided they should know because you care for them and would like them to get better, does not mean it is kind to them if you do. This is another very relevant law in the Universe: Everybody has their own choice and allowing them to have it (even if it is you), is the kindest thing you can do.

Even if that choice is to let their Body die and leave this earthly embodiment.

WHAT INVITATION FROM COMPLETE ALLOWANCE CAN ME AND MY BODY BE TO BE A COMPLETELY DIFFERENT POSSIBILITY?

You might be reading this book as someone recommended it to you or you "accidently" came across it, because you are looking to change up your life, which it will if you let it. Another possibility is that you are reading this book because someone you really care about deals with severe health issues. Please, promise me you won't force this information into their world because of what you have decided is the right thing for them to do. Start asking, "What allowance and invitation can I be?"

It will start to shift energy and allow you to be the source for kindness and change that is very much wished for on this planet. Would you consider being part of something greater? Would you consider letting the idea in that you are part of a miraculous Universe?

Would you be willing to not ever impose your opinion, point of view, on anybody, no matter how much you would like them to not suffer and no matter how much you would like them to change and be great?

Remember this please, if someone chooses to suffer the only

thing you can do is have allowance and kindness for their choice. That is TRUE CARING.

Would you be willing to know that this Universe desires you to have everything you desire and will always support any and all of your choices, even if it means you would like to die?

TRUE KINDNESS IS ALLOWING EVERY CHOICE!

Shame

Below is a copy of my very first coming out post on social media where I admitted I had cancer. This was big because, up until this point, I hadn't realized how deeply ashamed I was of the cancer I created. The comments were heartwarming and so nurturing and I once again was given evidence that the Universe has my back.

Dear Universe,

I am willing to be anything...
I am willing to do anything...
I am willing to lose everything...
I am willing to gain everything...
I am willing to lose everybody and...
I am willing to gain everybody...

day one week ago I went to the hospital.
For a while there's been a lump in my neck, yet nothing harmful they thought...

Until last week...
We have bad news for you Ms. Mevis: In the biopsy we took, we found thyroid cancer.
I will never forget that moment in that doctor's office... Where my being was about to check out and take off and I was like, "NO!" I am staying here whatever it takes.

While tears were running down my face the only word that came out of my mouth multiple times was FUCK! FUCK FUCK FUCK!!!

Last week was a rollercoaster. Trying to know what I know without buying into this reality of trauma and drama was quite interesting and challenging...

God knows I am beyond grateful that I was able to be facilitated in a class this weekend and have so many people around me who KNOW that there is something else possible than taking out my whole throat!

One of the things we spoke about during class was all the secrets that we keep to maintain our image. All the energy we have to use against ourself to maintain the lies we buy about ourselves and everybody around us, because deep down we decided that we are soooo wrong...

Sharing that I have cancer is one of the hardest things I have ever done...I strongly believed that if I would share this, that everybody would leave me...

Nobody would want to be with me anymore and I woulc
my business...
There is such a deep feeling of shame and failure, that I,
Access Consciousness Certified Facilitator, Yoga Teacher,
Person who empowers others...created cancer... and yet... I did!

Am I really willing to go beyond right and wrong?
Am I willing to gain and lose everything and everybody?
There is the space and freedom for choice...

Am I grateful for all the people around me that broke down
my barriers of receiving and by being willing to contribute
their kindness, time and magic...now and in the coming
period!

"Could this come to me with ease?" I wonder.

Maybe now is the time to really trust the Universe has my back!
To trust that there is always another possibility!
AND that we can change EVERYTHING, if we really choose it.

What else is possible now for me and my Body, that I didn't
think was possible that if I would allow the possibility to
show up, it would actualize another reality?

What if I don't have to hold up any lies or hide secrets
anymore?
What if in this reality I have cancer...but in my reality I just
have an identity crisis in my neck?

What would it take to just change this, because I want to
and choose it?

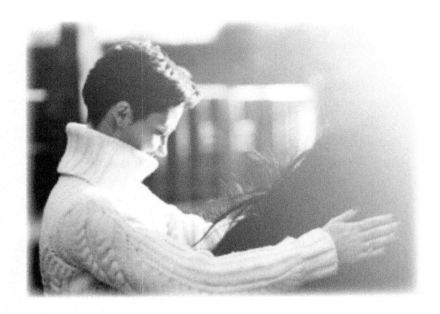

WHAT IF THE ONLY THINGS YOU CANNOT
CHANGE ARE THE THINGS YOU ARE NOT
WILLING TO BE AWARE OF?

What if *Anything* Can Change?

In the world of judgment there actually is no choice. Judgment only sticks you in the ongoing loop of trying to get it right. Well, that will be another totally weird thing to start embracing. What if you do not require to be right? It might be a beyond for you at this moment and yet I tell you it changed my life when my friend Dain Heer asked me one question.

I stood in front of the microphone in a big Access Consciousness® class asking a question on how to change my cancer. There were over 200 people in the room and the amount of energy that was changing and shifting and being exposed made me spin so hard that I had to hold the mic stand to not fall over. Looking at all sorts of choices I had been making not only this lifetime but through many lifetimes, my world got lighter. I got closer to me, at which moment I asked Dain, "How do I move on from here to change it?" He looked at me...and there it was, the question that knocked down all sorts of defense mechanisms that I built around truly knowing what I know and can be:

DO YOU REALLY WANT TO CHANGE IT, OR ARE YOU LOOKING TO BE RIGHT?

F*ck. Yes that, I was looking to be right...
My Body was crying of release, and do you know the beauty of every awareness that you allow yourself to have? It opens up space to make a different choice. The things that lock us into the impossibility of changing is our unwillingness to look at everything.

I do mean everything: the good, the bad, the beautiful and the ugly. Then, and only then, all the stuck beliefs and points of view that create the disease in the first place can leave your world, and your Body is set free to heal.

Your Body has a self-healing capacity that goes beyond anything you can cognitively imagine. You might have heard this story: that people miraculously heal from all sorts of things. Now be honest with yourself, do you know you can do that too? Or is this something that only certain privileged people can do?

IF I CAN DO IT, SO CAN YOU!

There is no reason in the world that would make anybody luckier, more privileged, more capable of changing their life around than you!

I am here to tell you that I will be your cheerleader. I will be empowering you to know that there is no wrong choice, not even dying. I will be empowering you to know what you know about what shows up in your Body and your life, and finally, I will be cheering you on front line to know that anything and everything you created and does not work anymore, you can out-create and change!

IF I DON'T NEED TO BE RIGHT, WHAT WOULD I CHOOSE?

After a few weeks of on and off fighting against myself, everybody's opinions, and my own judgments, this was one question that totally set me free to truly explore what my choices, my life, and my truth with all of this could be.

The only thing that gave me freedom out of this whole intense cocktail of fear, emotions, and feelings was being "okay" with dying. Truth be told, it took me 8 months before I chose to sit, alone, on my yoga pillow, having the courage to really receive the possibility of dying. Here I sat, silently, melting every barrier I thoroughly built around the idea of dying...first there was nothing and then there was a whole lot of tears.

After about 5 minutes of tears rolling down my face, it stopped. It was different; I was different; something truly changed. I allowed myself to receive the idea of dying and it gave me more peace than I could remember I ever had before.

It gave me a space to breathe; it gave me choice...

And this might sound extremely weird to a lot of people, but for you, if you are looking for this information, here it is...

THE MOMENT YOU ALLOW YOURSELF TO DIE, YOU OPEN UP TO THE UNIVERSE OF CHOICE!

The moment I allowed myself to die, I opened up to a whole Universe of Choice! You know why? Because now I was truly able to stop the fight. I was able to embrace the choice, and with that, the power and potency started to open.

You can start to look at what living means to you, how you like to create your life. You can start looking at what is valuable and real to YOU that makes life worth living.

The Universe always gives you what you have asked for.
It will not give you what you think you can handle... it will give you what you can truly handle.
And here is a whole new adventure of exploration about to start.

WHAT IF DYING IS NOT WRONG AND GIVES YOU THE FREEDOM TO TRULY LIVE?

From this space, my world started to relax...

Because I knew right from that moment, that there was something else available for me. A choice, a possibility that might not be available for everybody, but it was for me!
Not knowing how any of this was going to look like, I started one of the most expanding journeys of my life. "Okay Body, if you could choose whatever you wanted to choose, whether it was kick me out, whether it was die, whether it was taking the operation, whatever it was, what else is possible?"

I let go of control and that was the moment that everything

changed!

This came with a space of trust, allowance, and lack of fear of losing my Body.

We have choice, our Body has a choice, and we can change this together or not. From there on, everything changed and kept on changing, and to be honest, it is still expanding my life everyday.

It also came with the space for me to start asking.

WHAT IF NOTHING WE LEARNED ABOUT OUR BODY IS TRUE?

Now pause for a moment...

What have you learned about your Body?

Did you learn it was this magnificent potent creature that is able to create, out-create and change anything and everything? Or have you learned to always be careful to not kill it?

In this reality, we learned that we must protect our Body, that we must make sure our Body doesn't die. There is a lot of fear, as we are scared that something might happen to our Body.

Take your shots, eat healthy, be careful, don't get ill and so forth... and if there is something that could kill our bodies, let's cut it out.

I dare say that you have learned to protect your Body as well as 100% of the population on this planet. We must spend our life trying to not have our bodies die, to eventually...die... Not much living in this, is there?

All of this would be more surviving than thriving.

WHAT IF THERE IS A JOY OF EMBODIMENT AND COOPERATION WITH YOUR BODY AVAILABLE?

Is it at all real to you, that if we create, for example, a tumor, which will kill our Body, and we cut it out, without having a look at the point of view that created the tumor in the first place, that you will create a different way to die?

To me, it is and so I wish for everybody who is willing to know, to have this information.

To be very clear, it might be a great contribution to operate with regards to certain diseases and even get tumors cut out, YET you will have to look at the underlying point of view for it to be a sustainable change in your life.

My Body showed me a capacity for change and creation that is beyond this reality and what I have been told.

What I got to experience is that our Body is one of the most creative, healing, changing, miraculous beings that we get to create with and one of the greatest gifts of being alive.

It is exactly this fear and need for protection that keeps you from truly living and enjoying your life! It keeps you stuck in the circle of judgment and rightness to never ever be wrong.

WHAT IF YOU DON'T HAVE TO PROTECT YOUR BODY AGAINST DYING, YET ALL YOU HAVE TO DO IS TRULY CHOOSE TO LIVE?

Everything going on around the word cancer was extremely heavy to me. My Body invited me to become way more present with what is true for me, and I am inviting you to that space too! Are you willing to step into the miraculous being called YOU?

Who are you beyond every projection, expectation, and judgment that you are aware of?

Remember none of this must be yours unless you make it more real than you!

ARE YOU WILLING TO BE DIFFERENT?

I started to wonder...
Everything that is going on in this world is very factual. For example: Cancer will kill you.
It started to really sink in the moment when my wondrous puppy, Joy, ate a chocolate egg...
Immediately I went into the extreme upset (just like the *F*ck hospital you have got cancer* moment).
Within nanoseconds I downloaded, as the psychic SpongeBob we are, every point of view, every emotion, and every feeling about what it means when a dog eats chocolate.

I went into doubting what to do! Call the vet? Make her vomit? Do nothing?
I went into fear on what could happen! O my god, what if she does get ill? What if it will kill her?
I got super angry! Now this is something that you might not know, but for me was very helpful. I only get super angry when there is a lie present. It took me a bit (way too many hours) circling about in this wonderful cranky pants space when it suddenly came to me to ask a question to gain awareness.

I asked, "What is the lie here and what is Joy trying to make me aware of?"
And there it was – the big FAT lie that we all learned to

function from:

I cannot undo this, so I cannot change it!

WHAT IF FEAR, DOUBT AND ANGER ARE NOT REAL?

One of the lies we buy all the time is that we are powerless people, victims of circumstances, and completely unable to change anything and everything that happens to us. What my friend, if this is the greatest limitation that you have even been taught, programmed, and been entrained to believe?
Does any of this you are reading make you more Relaxed? More Peaceful? Maybe even Happier?
It is because deep down you know this to be true!

You know that there is a whole Universe available where you practice Magic? Where you have capacities to change everything in the speed of space and where you are a Powerhouse of Magnitude?

ARE YOU WILLING TO KNOW?

How does this work? Well, that is an exploration I started many years ago when I was DONE! Done suffering, done being unhappy, and moreover, done with being a victim of everything that showed up in my life.
I was a panic attack on legs..
Until I demanded it to change...

Access Consciousness® showed up in my life and from that point on, my life got greater every day.

Not because of the modality, but because of the empowerment to know what I know and the ongoing invitation to be more me! I learned tools and techniques to get to my power and to my unique brand of Magic. I learned that the energy I am willing to be in the world is an inspiration for other people to be more of them in the world, and that nature thrives on diversity! By now I am acknowledging that I have choices available that not everybody does, because of what I am willing to know. Would it be possible that you are reading this because you do too?

Back to the chocolate egg story with my dog... Beyond the doubt, fear, and anger was me as a possibility.

What did I truly know?

HOW MUCH DO WE USE FACTS OF DRAMA FROM THIS REALITY AS A WAY TO TURN DOWN THE MAGIC AND CHANGE WE CAN CREATE?

I knew that my dog was fine, and I also knew that we could change everything.
Peace restored, we made the choice to be great and to use the tools I had available. We fell a sleep together while I was holding her Body running beautiful healing energies.

Not in one single way could it be noted that she ate chocolate; it was almost like it never happened. It was almost like we just changed it.
And truth be told, I am in love with all these animals that are always willing to show up as greater and invite us to be greater too!
How many of these miracle workers do you have around you,

that you might have never even acknowledged?

WHAT IF YOU STARTED TO LOOK AT EVERYTHING BEYOND THE JUDGMENT OF IT?

What if this could be a key that sets us free? It does not matter whether it is about a disease that you have going on, or a dog that ate chocolate, or money that you lost, or anything else in your life that seems to be bad and awful.

Would it be possible that you get to show up with way more power and possibilities than you ever thought you had available?
Now be aware! This is not normal and there will be very few people that are able to see it this way! As I said, you might have choices, magic, and possibilities available that are only for the ones that are looking for it!

"The ones that don't believe in magic will never find it." – Roald Dahl
"The ones that do will be amazed over and over again!" – Saskia Mevis

WHAT IF NOTHING ANYONE SAYS MUST BE TRUE FOR YOU? WHAT IS YOUR REALITY WITH THIS?

Did I experience fear of dying? Yes!
Did I resist and avoid knowing whether my Body wanted the operation? Yes!
Did I experience very strong panic attacks where it felt like I could not swallow anymore? Yes...
Did I have moments where I doubted any other possibilities in my world? Absolutely!
Was I the effect of other people projecting their feelings at

me? Yes. Some moments I had no clue what was mine or what I perceived around me...
BUT
Did I sleep well and have the willingness to move forward? ABSOLUTELY!

Did I experience a massive support from people and forces beyond words having my back? HOLY FUCK YES!
Did I get closer and closer to the Peace and the Potency that the Universe really will have my back, even if it doesn't look like the way I think it should? TOTALLY!

IF I WOULD BE WILLING TO LOSE EVERYTHING, INCLUDING MY LIFE... WHAT POSSIBILITIES COULD SHOW UP?

Man, am I grateful for the people in my life that KNOW!
The almost overwhelming support in Energies
The Empowering words
The Gifted sessions
The Contributions to my Body and Being
The people I can call at any time when I just totally seem to lose it just because I buy into the reality of having cancer...

I would like to mention that for my family it has been a very bumpy ride. It was very difficult for them to see me make choices that they were not comfortable with.

I am not going to make this prettier than it was. I created some serious upset in my parents' world and while I did not lose any minute of sleep over all of this, they did.
For them it would have been way easier to see me make the traditional choices, and yet I just could not. For them, it was

like losing their daughter repeatedly as I did not make those choices.

I think that was one of the hardest things to deal with – how other people dealt with it. Because in case you didn't know, thyroid cancer is normally very "easily treated" with an operation where they cut open your throat, they take out your thyroid, take out your lymph, and they put you five days in radioactive isolation. Nobody talks about how your thyroid is one of the most magical glands in your Body that basically supports all your organs!

The reason why I am sharing this is you might find people around you who aren't cheering you on for your choices to be different. Yet just know, it is their way of caring for you. It is their way of proving themselves that they care. It is all we ever learn about caring. That in order to care for someone else you have to be willing give yourself and your peace up, rather than allowing themselves to have allowance for all choices which is true caring, which nobody taught us. Receiving the gift of their caring without having to comply to their reality might be a challenge, but I know YOU GOT THIS, as did I, no matter how uncomfortable it may seem and get.

WHAT IF TRUE CARING MEANS ALLOWING EVERYBODY THEIR OWN CHOICE AND SUPPORTING THAT?

"How are you?"
This is a question I have been asked many times a day... since I have been diagnosed as "ill".
I know that this is the way for people to let me know that they care.

I also know that many times this question comes with a certain expectation, judgment, even a projection...

In the beginning, it was difficult for me. I was willing to give up my trust, my allowance, my magic, my possibility and my gratitude because I knew other people were not able to understand it. I was not willing to freak them out, offend them, or scare them away with my reality.

I realized that I am so aware of the energy behind every question that I jump into all universes to answer and actually BE the expected and projected response...which is different every time.

"I am good!"
"Up and Down...."
"Takes too long..."
"I am done and it changes too slow..."
"I just keep going; all will be good."
"I am very tired, because my Body works so hard!"
"I trust that it will work out fine..."

These are some of the answers that I watch myself merge into...depending on who is asking the question.

How are you? *What does this even mean?* I've asked myself many times.

Very smooth and so cute, yet not so bright...you know why not? Because while being busy answering to all of those asked and unasked questions, I forgot what is actually going on for me... What is true for me?

Almost like I hid it in such a way that I could not find it anymore myself.

My Body and I are exploring a new way of being together and

creating together that is beyond words and different every day. I am not good, not bad, not sick and not better!
Truly what else is possible if we are willing to go beyond every shape shifting that we do to be received by others?

ARE YOU WILLING TO CREATE A NEW REALITY WITH YOUR BODY?

After about 2 years I was on my way for a walk with my friend when we started to talk about my idea of writing a book. She was thrilled and told me that it was such a gift to see how I dealt with it. I asked her what she experienced, and this is what she said and asked me.

Normally when people get ill, they think, "O my god! I am ill!" and they go into survival mode. You chose another space. You went from the space of "I got this" and "How does it get better than this?"

"How can this contribute to me?" For the outside world you are not ill. You are just phenomenal.

The thing I had been wondering was how to deal with you.

There is the point of view that I must show people that I care, by asking them how they are doing, while at the same time not wanting to bring it up all the time.

My question is, "How do I be with people that are ill?"

This is an interesting question to address, because you might totally get it, or you might get extremely offended with what I am about to write here.

We make interaction with other people difficult because of all the expectations, judgments, and projections we put on it. What if we could make it easy?

What if you could just ask the person: "Hey, I truly hope you know I care for you and also can you please tell me what way of dealing with it contributes the most to you?"

If you would have asked me that question, I would have told you that I know you care and that you don't ever have to prove this to me. Being the space of allowance for whatever I choose and supporting that has been the greatest gift to me.

Know some people really love the attention. There are many people that create diseases from the value of attention. Now what if this is not wrong either? But a great gift to acknowledge and be in allowance with? It makes it easier for you to deal with and it gives them the space to choose something different.

WHAT IF YOU NEVER HAVE TO PROVE YOU CARE?

Your *Body*

To read on, you must for a second know that your Body is not just a piece of flesh at your disposal.

Your Body is an organism made from the same substance as the Earth. It has its own consciousness. You have two choices on this matter. Are you choosing to create with it and see it as your best friend? Or are you going to keep dismissing it, as if it is not valuable at all? I understand due to upbringing, culture and religion the Body has always been seen as less than... but what if that, again, is a massive lie? What if your Body is a true GIFT?

WHAT IF YOU WOULD START TO SEE YOUR BODY AS YOUR PARTNER IN CRIME?

One morning in the shower I held my Body, touched my neck

and asked:

"Sweet beautiful wonderful Body, what else is possible for us, that we didn't think was possible, that if we would allow the possibility to show up, would actualize a completely different reality?

I will let go of control and please create whatever you desire to create: Healing, Operation, or even Death...if there is no right or wrong, I will not have to fight for or against anything.

What else is possible then?"

Two hours later I was booked on a plane to Thailand where I received an alternative treatment that got arranged with more ease than I ever experienced in my life before.

Did I know that it would work? Nope!

Did I know that whatever showed up I would keep following the lightness and taking the stepping stones? Yes!

Did I know that I would be and do whatever it took to change this and learn to trust even more what I know and that the Universe has my back? HELL TO THE YES!!!

So if you would not have to buy into this reality, but you get to create your own, where there is Ease and Joy no matter what shows up?

WHAT IF THERE IS MAGIC AROUND EVERY CORNER IN EVERY MOMENT?

What is more relevant to you: Acknowledging the choices that you make now? Or making yourself wrong for the choices that you didn't make in the past? I call that an anchor point. We have a choice that we did or did not make in the past, and we make that an anchor point for wrongness. So whatever you create now, whatever you choose now, no matter how great your life will get, you will always go back to that anchor point. Because then you know you can always make yourself wrong. If only you would have chosen that then, then your great life would have shown up way earlier.

Going to the wrongness of you is always a choice. Are you willing to acknowledge that it's a choice, and it's a very comfortable choice? Rather than making the uncomfortable choice, which would mean you refuse to go to the wrongness of you.

How much would your life change if you would right now refuse to go to the wrongness of you?

Ponder for a minute. If just for today, there would be no right choice and no wrong choice, what would be possible?

HOW FUN WOULD YOUR LIFE BE?

What if there is always a beautiful energy underneath it all and that everything is the opposite of what it appears to be? This song showed up in my world while I was teaching my last yoga class before my trip and for me it is the Universe talking to me!

The power of love is here now
The power of now is here now
The power of you and me is here
To create magic on earth

Let the water wash away your tears
Let the fire burn away your fears
Let the wind blow into your life such faith and trust, oh

Let the earth hold you, take care of you and nurture you
- Alexia Chellun[1]

ARE YOU RECEIVING YOUR BODY AS THE GIFT IT TRULY IS?

By following the energy, I ended up in a private clinic in Thailand.
I now know why it wasn't light to just get operated on and to get everything removed.
It simply is not my way...
Apart from the fact that removing the tumors including very important glands like lymph and thyroid is a very invasive operation, there is so much more going on energetically underneath this all!

All along I have been asking for clarity and contribution and more and more all pieces of the puzzle fell into place. What I created with my Body is not something that happened to me... It is something that came up because I was ready to face it and change it all right now!

YOU ARE NOT BROKEN!

"What strengths am I not acknowledging?"
Strength is the place where you cannot be broken....

At some point, huge awareness hit me! Tears running down my face... When I am me... I am whole... that world where I am willing to be me in communion with everything...

1 The Power is Here Now, by Alexia Chellun, from the album *Just Before I Sleep*, (P)&(C)2018

The other world...the world where there is the lump...where there is the cancer I believed that I was broken....That for some reason my Body was broken and wrong...

The thing with awareness is, you get it when you get it...

If there is a hidden unseen point of view that you are broken... you do not have all of you, you have not acknowledged that strength of you...

AND remember your point of view creates your reality!

For a long time I tried to fix myself and my Body. About one and half years down the road, I was still fixing it. It got subtle over time, but I was still functioning form the space that there was something wrong.

Suddenly it got to me, I was waiting...For example, I was not going to get a puppy until the cancer was gone. There the awareness was: this is bullshit. So now I'm going to wait to live until I stop dying?

WHAT HAVE I DECIDED IS WRONG ABOUT ME, THAT IS ACTUALLY STRONG ABOUT ME?

Where do we still make ourselves wrong and believe we are broken so we can fit into the trauma and drama of this reality? What if we have the choice to invite a completely different awareness about everything we choose and create? Even if it is uncomfortable?

Because yes, that is what it will be with (many) moments.

Yet if you are willing to look at everything, you know what? You can change ANYTHING!

THE THINGS YOU ARE NOT WILLING TO LOOK AT STICK YOU IN THE WORLD OF LIMITATION AND UNHAPPINESS.

Living

Since I realized that I was creating my way of escaping this life and reality by killing my Body, I demanded that to change!

I started asking: What would it take for me to truly live?
You know this? Where are you looking for the joy and enthusiasm that seems nowhere to be found?
That was my life for a long time.... based on lies and points of view that were not even mine!

Are you creating your life based on your reality and commitment to YOU?
Or are you having this backdoor where you allow yourself to leave all the time?
(literally and energetically)

What would show up if we would collectively commit to our life and our reality?

My life keeps expanding, my Body keeps amazing me, my world(s) keep on growing and in the meanwhile, insanity melts more and more out of my world and out of this beautiful Planet!

Embracing the perfect in the imperfect taught me how stuck we are in pictures of ourselves, our lives, our relationships, our bodies, our business and well...everything around us... What if we would choose the POWER of PRESENCE in every moment and keep on MELTING into the POWER, POTENCY MAGIC and MYSTERIES, KINDNESS and CARING that becomes more and more available every day?

I know I am not perfect and never will be, but as a very inspiring person once said to me, you are great today and you will be greater tomorrow!

For our bodies to truly change in a miraculous way we have to let go of as many points of view as we can (if not all of them! ☺)

WHAT WOULD IT TAKE TO TRULY LIVE?

How much are you trained to judge your Body? How much are you judging your Body all the time?

We are raised, entrained, programmed, and cultivated to function from the space of judgment. What is judgment? It is the right and wrong side about everything and anything.

It means that whatever happens in your life, or on a smaller scale, during your day, will be categorized. It either goes into the "this is good" pile or the "this is bad and should not have happened" pile.

It makes sure that you never enter the Magic space where you can receive everything with a sense of gratitude.

You can imagine that cancer, or any other disease, within seconds goes to the "this is bad and should never have happened" pile.

And exactly that is the space where you must start fighting, you must make it wrong, you have to go to the blame and shame. What if instead for whatever is going on in your world, you could go to the space of gratitude?

Gratitude is one of the most healing and generative
energies in the world!

I can imagine that being grateful for intense and sad things in your world is a major stretch. Believe me, I know, and I have been there. That is why I would like you to start cultivating gratitude for you. For the wonderful person you are. Start looking at you as if you are a gift to the world.

ARE YOU GRATEFUL FOR YOU?

Only if you can start to see the gift that you be, will there be relaxation for the things that show up. From this place on, you can start cultivating gratitude for the wonderful Body that you chose and created, no matter what is going on in your Body at this exact moment. Allow yourself to drop all defense mechanisms and receive the energy of gratitude. Acknowledge that no matter how hard it is, you have been part of creating what showed up now. You might have difficulties going there, but believe me, when you do, you open up to one of the greatest powers there is. When you can go to the gratitude for you and for everything that shows up in your world, you have the power to shift, change and rearrange everything based on that gratitude.

You know what the secret is? When you have gratitude for your disease, condition, or anything else in your world, it means that nothing is wrong aka there is no judgment about it. The judgment creates the need for it to change. In the space of gratitude, it does not HAVE to change. From here, with no need to change it, you can change everything! The key is no judgment and no need for it to be different!

WHAT IF GRATITUDE IS THE KEY TO CHANGE EVERYTHING?

One of the most important things is to get out of reaction.
We start fighting against the cancer, against the disease, and exactly that energy will keep you from the choice to change it.
To be really honest, it took quite a while for me to really be in total allowance. The first year it was mostly being in acceptance. Which means, it is wrong but okay...There is still the need for it to change because otherwise you are wrong. Only when it all is gone and I have the proof of this, will my life be right again.

THE NEED TO BE RIGHT TAKES AWAY YOUR CHOICE TO BE FREE!

What if everything, that shows up in your Body is an awareness and not something that needs to be fixed, but something that you could receive?
What if there would be no expectation that it goes away? I know you would rather vomit than linger in the idea of something that you have made wrong about your Body never changing; this is our inherent need to fix everything.

Have you acknowledged that you chose your Body; you created your Body?

You are the one having this Body! So, basically everywhere where you have a point of view about how your Body shows up, how your Body looks, how your Body acts, how your Body is not changing or changes, is where you make your choice for your Body to be wrong! It will make you infinitely suffer your Body and your embodiment.

MAKING YOUR BODY WRONG MAKES YOU SUFFER THROUGH LIFE INDEFINITELY!

One of the most remarkable stories is the one of my lump.

There had been a lump in my neck for years, even before I had the sense of going to the doctor it had been there. You could see it, you could feel it and to be clear, the lump was wrong, it was ugly, and it just had to go...

After getting more and more present with my Body and a conversation with my Thai doctor, I realized that this lump was what saved my life. It kept the cancer from spreading through my whole Body.

The moment I realised the lump was what kept me from dying, my whole world shifted into gratitude for my Body. Can you imagine that something in your Body, no matter what it is, that you have made extremely wrong, would be a GIFT? Would there be a possibility that your wonderful Body knows what it is doing?

We do this with everything in our lives. We have many judgments about so many things that show up in our bodies, show up in our relationships, show up in our business, in our money, in our lives, in our everything. What if we would start asking: "What is the gift here?" You could start to acknowledge that there is a beautiful energy underneath it all. This is where the journey of receiving starts.

Maybe the lump never leaves and what if that's okay?! For me, it's an everyday reminder to receive it all.

YOUR BODY IS NOT MADE TO SELF-DESTRUCT; IT IS MADE TO HEAL!

This raised the question: What if it doesn't have to go away? Would I be okay? Would I even be Happy?

My Body over the years has shown amazing results on all levels and very well above average vitality. Am I really going to let a lump that saved my life and gave me the choice to truly live make my life wrong? Or am I going to linger in the gratitude of this invitation to more living?

Because here is another little secret to be told. If I would have to do it all over again, I would not have changed a thing. The cancer has turned out to be one of the greatest gifts that still keeps on expanding my awareness beyond the limited parameters of this world.

What I realized was that our bodies are our greatest guide to consciousness.

We have so many points of view and stuff going on in our heads. Never will this bring you to peace. Because be honest, if you could figure life out with your head, would you not already have done it?

Your Body KNOWS the way to Consciousness; it knows the way to Ease and Joy!

It's basically like a shortcut.

*Can you imagine that nothing in your Body needs to be fixed?
It only desires to be received!*

WHAT IF YOUR BODY IS A GUIDE TO CONSCIOUSNESS?

Allowing
Yourself to Die!

Before I wrote about how I had to get to the space of allowance with my choices, I had to give myself complete choice, even if that meant I would die.

Here is the thing: As long as you fight against death, you will be controlled by death.

I realized more than ever before that EVERYTHING we avoid or hide because we are not willing to look at it...will stick us... it is the ONLY thing that will stick us and keep us from truly being FREE!

After 8 months of having the concept of cancer living in my Body, I was TRULY willing to be present with the possibility of dying...

The possibility of leaving my Body...

It was only a few small single minutes in which tears were pouring down my face, but it changed my life forever...

And I knew it... I knew I was avoiding it... and at the same time I did not...if you get what I mean...Your head thinks it is present while you make up enough brainfood to not ever really receive what is going on for you.

For 8 months I avoided it in the most elegant way possible... until I didn't anymore...

Are you done avoiding?

WHEN YOU ARE WILLING TO ACKNOWLEDGE YOU ARE DYING, YOU HAVE THE CHOICE TO TRULY LIVE.

Was this period always easy for me?

No absolutely not!

I have been very uncomfortable and very intense...I have lost my patience. I have been angry. I have been extremely frustrated and sad. Yet looking back on it, it all has been with a sense of ease!

Truth be told (and I know this is hard for the people who care about me)...

I did not lose one minute of sleep on this whole creation.

One of the magical things that I have experienced, and I would like you to get a sense of, is that in the space of consciousness there is no stress available. Stress is based on the lie that you are subject to and victim of what happens to you. When you start to acknowledge the enormous amount of power and potency you have for creation, you open a completely different possibility. Beyond stress there is a sense of relaxation with whatever shows up in your life.

IT WON'T BE EASY BUT IT CAN STILL BE WITH A LOT OF EASE!

The acknowledgement that the cancer was something I created myself, that I was secretly choosing to die, and that I also had the choice in every moment how to move on from here, brought me ease...and a sense of peace with all of it... the good, the bad, the ugly... all with a sense of allowance and knowing that nothing had to be fixed.
I only had to choose what was real and true for me!

It was exactly that which inspired me to keep going...to keep choosing to become greater in every moment! I kept and keep on asking for Consciousness to show me the way literally in every 10 seconds and allowing my Body to override me.
I chose and choose to keep on asking questions and trust the choices I make are creating the greatest future for me, my Body, and eventually, the Planet.

What would it take for you to move forward with your Body reaching for more consciousness?
What would it take to have Ease, Joy, Glory, and Clarity with what is Real and True for you?
What would it take to not be the effect of anything or anybody else that you are aware of and think is bigger or greater than you and your knowing?

WHAT WOULD IT TAKE TO CREATE A LIFE THAT INSPIRES YOU?

What turns your Body on?

Where have you given up on creating with your Body, because you tried to get it right and you couldn't?

Here's the newsflash!

You will never create your Body right!

Yet... you can create extraordinarily with your Body!

WHAT CAN YOU BE TO BE ENERGETICALLY CONGRUENT WITH YOUR BODY'S EXTRA-ORDINARY POSSIBILITIES?

Pondering about receiving...

How much have you secretly decided that receiving is not real?

Working hard is real...

Suffering is real...

Force is real...

Just being and allowing everything to be Magic, Ease, Joy and Exuberant Expression of Life and Abundance is not anything close to what we have been taught...

We have many ideas on what receiving is, how it looks, and what it means.

What if I tell you that honestly none of that is true?

Receiving seems so obvious, but what if it isn't?

What if receiving has many more shapes, forms, and possibilities than we allow?

Yes! Receiving seems most of the time materialized but what if most of it happens energetically?

The thing is, we only learn the concept of receiving, which is very limiting. It is based on judgment, definition, and expectation.

Can you imagine that there is another possibility?

When I found that out, I was so excited!
Like a whole new world opened for me, a world that I always knew was there and never seemed to have access to, until I did!

Receiving always has a sense of peace and ease to it! No matter how hard, no matter how intense, no matter how difficult...
Nothing to save, nothing to change, nothing to fix!
True receiving means nothing is wrong EVER!
What have you made so wrong about you that you refuse to receive it?

IS IT TIME TO START RECEIVING ALL OF YOU?

Healing

This reality is not based on trust and knowing. It is based on drama and trauma. We seem to be addicted to fearing the worst-case scenario. We seem to thrive on shit that locks us out of happiness and stick ourselves with the belief that happiness is not real.

Getting back to the psychic SpongeBob you are...can you imagine that it is really easy to buy a gram of drama, doubt, and fear on about every corner of everybody's head? Might it at all be real to you that you don't HAVE TO buy into drama that is not YOURS?

One day, on my way to the clinic, it came to me... I have been so present with following my knowing all the way up here.... if it is not ease and spacious, it is not my Body's, because she does not talk to me like this. I am just aware of shitloads around this subject, points of view, perceptions and all sorts of people, energies, demons, entities, call them whatever you want.

The thing is that these moments will circle you to a place where you don't really like to hang out. It is the space of doubt. The problem with doubt is that you must give up your reality and your Magic in order to make it real.

So please start realizing that just like fear, doubt is also never real...

Every time I realize this, my whole Body surrenders.

DOUBT KILLS THE FOUNDATION OF THE CHANGE AND MAGIC YOU CREATED!

What are you choosing?

Are you choosing for you?

Are you choosing to heal your Body being the Magic you truly be?

What else is truly possible if we would refuse to go into any form of trauma and drama and you're willing to know that there's always another possibility for more joy and more of YOU?

ARE YOU CHOOSING TO HEAL?

What truly inspires you?

What makes you excited to wake up in the morning and create your life?

What is that thing in the whole wide World that would make you willing to BE and DO EVERYTHING that is required for it to be created?

Creating a disease in your Body is not very difficult; it comes with your willingness to give up and die out of your caged life...

Healing is a whole different ball game.

It requires you to have true vulnerability. The willingness to look at everything and keep on choosing beyond. It requires you to have the willingness to become aware of what is truly going on in your world and in the world.

It asks from you that you BE MORE of YOU!

HEALING IS THE SIDE EFFECT OF BECOMING MORE CONSCIOUS!

What is Consciousness? It is the inclusion of EVERYTHING without any judgment. It is the embodiment of ALLOWANCE for everything that shows up in your world and the World.

It is the willingness to take full responsibility of stepping up to creating your life without having anything or anybody to blame...

It means reaching to become greater every moment of every day as you are reaching to be the greatest you can be...

Not according to the measures of this reality, but to the resources that are so far beyond this reality that they are totally dismissed...

What would it take for us to be INSPIRED?

Ponder for a moment what the world would look like if we would all be INSPIRED by life?

What future would we all create if we would ask the infinite Universe, our Bodies, and every conscious element to show us how much greater things could become in order to get really inspirational?

Would we be willing to ask for WAY greater?!

For me, this has been the adventure and it still is....if we would claim, own and acknowledge that we are all unique creatures that came here with the capacity to create ongoing Magic and Miracles, then truly what else is possible for the evolution of human kind?

WHAT IF ONE OF OUR GREATEST CAPACITIES IS TO ASK FOR GREATNESS?

It takes time to be present with what your Body is showing you instead of jumping to conclusions.
If you have decided that vulnerability is a weakness, you will continue to build barriers to not acknowledge what is possible with the changes.
Vulnerability is the path to possibilities and potency!

We can no longer afford to not be space. In contraction there are only judgments and we do not allow ease and vulnerability... then we start hurting ourselves literally and figuratively, and we move away from the possibilities again. In this contraction everything becomes personal and we do not allow ourselves to be the LEADER OF CONSCIOUSNESS.

Space is energy and the infiniteness that you are in all directions... in space you can't hold points of view and that's Magic! Then you can move to your greatness, and you have choice!
So what would it take to make space one of the most valuable things in your life? Not just one day... but every day.

YOU who show up every day and contribute to creating a LIGHTER WORLD!
YOU, the MAGICIAN that you are!
YOU, the BEACON OF LIFE that you are!

What can you receive from Consciousness in this adventure? How much ease are you willing to receive?

And what if in this receiving, in this ease and in this space you and your Body have choice and you can co-create? What if that's the Magic to possibilities you never thought was possible...

For you, for others, for creating a lighter world, a different reality...?

What can you facilitate now without being its effect any longer and can you SHINE as BRIGHT as you truly are?!

It's time to step up and keep going! BE the BEACON OF LIFE... BE the POSSIBILITY!

IS LIFE WORTH LIVING WITHOUT BEING ABLE TO BE WHO YOU TRULY ARE?

Creating with Your Body, the Earth, and the Future

From this point on, what else do you have available to choose? What if this is just the beginning of a completely different reality with bodies and your Body in particular?

Creation is not something that you learn when you're young. You learn to control you, to judge you; you learn to put things in linear patterns, but you do not learn the Magic of creation. And really, one of the basic things that you got to get is in order to create with anybody or anything, you must be beyond judgment, because judgment is the killer of creation.

Is receiving valued in this world? No!
Is relaxation valued in this world? No!

Is ease valued in this world? No!

WHAT WOULD IT TAKE TO OPEN TO THE SPACE OF RELAXATION WHERE TRUE CREATION IS AVAILABLE?

If you'd like to hold on to the stress with your Body, if you'd like to hold on to the judgment of your Body, if you'd like to hold on to the limited points of view that you're avoiding and defending to never be as great as you truly can be, then please stay away from anything that will gain more consciousness.

If you desire something different, I invite you to listen to the Exercise below and truly surrender beyond all control you have ever learned.

 www.saskiamevis.com/choosetolive

YOUR BODY IS A GIFT!

One of the most underestimated, dismissed and maybe even unknown phenomena is your Body's consciousness. Your Body is not just a piece of flesh...It is a conscious element, and it knows...A LOT!

Every lie, every judgment, every projection that you take on (things that are basically not true for you) shows up in your Body as something that is solid and unchangeable. Every disease is information that desires to be received.

When you start living, speaking, and embodying your truth, your Body will start melting and exposing more and more information to you. Can you imagine that my greatest changes on my way to consciousness came from information that my Body showed me? Your Body is a library of knowledge collected throughout lifetimes and it is up to you to acknowledge it. Will you start receiving this or will you keep rejecting it?

Is it at all real to you that your Body might be holding some keys to magic?

Your Body is a powerhouse, and it has so much to show you and share with you!

ARE YOU BRAVE ENOUGH TO GIVE YOUR BODY THE LEAD?

Would you value yourself enough to create greater for yourself and the world?

Every different choice you make for your Body creates a different future for the planet.

Would you be willing to truly value the difference, the gift and the possibility you be for this planet and for the future?

You choosing to be different with your Body means being different with the Earth. It is what creates something different with every choice you make to nurture your Body into greater. When you nurture your Body into something greater you are adding to the sustainable future of the planet. What if your Body is like a tree? You can kill it and you can recycle it. Your Body comes from the Earth and will go back to the Earth. It is literally made out of the same substance. It will be ever changing and ever evolving yet never going to be lost. Your Body is one, or as I call it, in communion, with the planet. Unfortunately, most of the time we control it out of communion.

What can you receive from your Body and create with it while you have it? Bodies invite you to those awarenesses where you have a different choice that you've not allowed yourself to have yet.

Gary Douglas once said and I thought it was brilliant; "You can recycle until hell freezes over, but that's not going to save the world." In other words, acknowledging your Body as part of the planet is the key to creating a thriving planet.

YOU AND YOUR CHOICES ARE RELEVANT FOR THE FUTURE OF THE PLANET!

At the end of this book, you might be happy, sad, empowered, angry, relaxed or many other things if not all at the same time. You might love me and what I have put out here; you might hate me and think this is absolutely ridiculous. You might want to absolutely know more, or you might not ever revisit this information ever again.

And you know what? All of that is great!

There is no right way or wrong way to receive this and there is no right way to live with and through disease.

What is relevant is that I wrote it down. Here is what I know about it...in the world... ready to be found by those who are looking for this.

Ready to empower you to know what you know!

Imagine that only one person picks up this book and changes his or her whole life...

Would it be worth writing it down? You might think no...

Here is where I beg to differ.

The fact is that each and every single person that chooses more of them contributes to everybody else having a greater future available.

My next question for you would be, What is it that you know

that wants to be heard in the world?

Often disease ground is where we are not totally willing to have our own reality, including all the Magic, Power and Possibilities that we truly be. What if you starting to embrace that not only changes the trajectory of your life and Body, but also the trajectory for the whole world and everybody that you are inviting to that? ☺

WHAT DO YOU DARE NOT SAY THAT, IF YOU WOULD DARE TO SAY IT, WOULD ALTER REALITIES?

I have been judged enormously!

And you most likely will be too. Don't ever dim yourself and your knowing down for that. This is what we've been doing for way too long. We've been saying, "You must be right, and you must know more than me," for all of our lives. Now it's time say something different!

"No, you're not right; you're not correct. I have a different reality. I know that you don't have a choice available to choose to change this, but I have!"

That's one of the other things you know...you have choice. When you're reading this, you have a choice available that not everybody has. When you start claiming, owning, and acknowledging this, you can be the inspiration for people who not yet have that choice available. Instead of trying to dim yourself down, make yourself ill, or kill yourself, turn it up and don't mind the people that don't desire to have it.

Do not try to force this point of view or this possibility onto people. Be the invitation and be willing to let them have their point of view, because that's one of the most important things. Remember we live in a free will Universe, and everybody has the right to their own choice.

LET YOURSELF BE JUDGED; IT IS NOT REAL OR RELEVANT!

Can you perceive that if I would have had the operation yet I still wanted to die, that I would have created something else to die?

What we often do is focus on the symptoms to go away and, for example, cut out tumors as soon as possible. My point of view is that without looking at the energy underneath the cancer or any other disease, you can cut it out or remove the symptoms, but you will create a different kind of cancer or disease, or you will just crash your car against a tree and die. My point is that if you are determined to die, you will die.

For the record and as a disclaimer, and for everything else: I'm not saying do not operate. I'm not saying do not take treatment. Take all of that, if you desire. Do everything that what works for you. It just didn't work for me. In addition, to whatever treatment you're choosing, please, please, please, please look at the energy and the points of view that are underneath. Otherwise, you will keep creating and generating it in a different way in a different form, and then you're still not living.

EVERY DEATH IS A (UN)CONSCIOUS CHOICE.

Beyond Your *Body*

Do you know that you are an infinite being? Do you know that if you would walk off the cliff and lose your Body that you're still there?

Now this is where it becomes deep!

It basically means you are an infinite being; you have always been and you will always be. There is no end to you and there are no limitations.

This gave me freedom to know that me as an infinite being would always be, and always will be, and that everything else is co-creation with the Earth, my Body, and Possibilities.

DO YOU KNOW THAT YOU ARE AN INFINITE BEING?

One of the greatest gifts is Access Consciousness® being in my life far before I got diagnosed.

For about 7 years, I have been committing to Consciousness in my life. The elegance and timing of Consciousness is not like anything I have ever seen before. I became a certified facilitator in August 2019, and I was diagnosed with cancer in October 2019. It was exactly what I required to live and be with all of this in the way I have been choosing. The elegance and timing of Consciousness is magical!

CONSCIOUSNESS GIFTS YOU POSSIBILITIES WHEN THIS REALITY SAYS THERE ARE NONE...

So there is one thing I KNOW more than anything else...

The Universe is tilting, shifting, and changing and our choices are what creates that, when we are totally willing to acknowledge our energetic capacities and we are willing to keep choosing for more and greater beyond judgment, trauma, drama and everything else that will limit you and keep you away from the space and the Freedom of you!

It is now your choice. It is not my choice. It is not the choice "other people" make...

When I look at my Body the shifts and changes it made and is making, there is no other explanation than that we are part of something Greater, something big, something that will have your back never mind how much you are ignoring and even fighting it!

Now is the time that avoiding possibilities is going to exhaust you, because NOW IS THE TIME TO LEAP!

Are you done avoiding the brighter, greatest future, while

getting exhausted?

Let's just change tracks, let's go and BE the MAGIC we truly BE!

Will you please acknowledge that every choice you make will create and invite something that is so far beyond this reality that you have no clue how to give words to it, yet the energy is becoming clearer with every step you have to courage to take? I am grateful. Are you too?

IS WHAT YOU KNOW VALUABLE?

You are never alone. There are always people that have your back and Consciousness has your back. There is nothing that is stronger than that!

One of the most valuable things that I would like you to get out of this book is the fact that you can create anything and everything and you can change anything and everything into greater!

YOU CAN CHANGE EVERYTHING!

Afterword

THE UNIVERSE DESIRES TO HAVE YOUR BACK!

Whether you are willing to receive that is up to you!

No matter in what area of your life you are stuck, there is ALWAYS another possibility! A possibility to create the life you desire. I'm sure you'll be amazed with your own power and potency when you start acknowledging the gift you truly are.

Trust me. I know. I've been there. I have come a long, beautiful way and here I am committed to spreading more Consciousness on this planet as an Access Consciousness® Certified Facilitator, but more importantly as ME!

I truly wonder what else is possible for YOU, beyond what you ever imagined?

What would it take for all of us, to keep choosing more in every moment and create greater possibilities for our lives, living AND the future of our beautiful planet?

What if you don't have to create cancer to leave your Body? What if you would start to live from the free will universe, where you have infinite possibilities and infinite choice in every moment? What if you can choose to live or die without suffering?

WHAT IF YOU CAN LIVE WITH EASE AND DIE WITH EASE?

I desire you to acknowledge Consciousness for its elegance and it's absolute determination, because consciousness is like no other man, no other woman, no other thing that you've ever seen before. Consciousness will find its way through each and every limitation. Consciousness will find its way for you, as you, through you, as you are willing to allow it and choose it. There is nothing that has your back more than consciousness. Melt into that. Melt your Body into that space.

We facilitate by being on the planet and that might sound awesome; "I'm facilitating consciousness all the time". But do you really get it? Do you receive how light and true that is for you?

YOUR CHOICE CREATES WHAT SHOWS UP IN YOUR WORLD.

In this lifetime, this reality is a boxed construct. You are born, you have your life, and then you die. That's it! I played with the question, 'what happens when I die?' and I realized that I locked up many points of view about death, about life, about what it means, and about what it doesn't mean, and that not being real and true for me, while making them real and true. Now I'm here in a different space in a different time to start claiming, owning, and acknowledging that there has been a lot of lies that kept me locked into the construct of this reality and death and life.

Sometimes it is so easy to buy into the point of view 'let me just die, because this world is going to hell anyway', where we use Death and Dying as a sweet escape in case it doesn't work out. This point of view, my dear friends, is not real nor true. It is impelled on us!

Is now the time to let go of having life as the sweet escape for death and death as the sweet escape for life so you never have to choose either of them?

We think it's all about life. That's the hook. If we would truly live, we would not be captured in the lies of death and life. We often refuse to truly live so that we can be stuck in death and life.

One of my favourite questions I started to play with is 'What would it take for me to truly live with this embodiment?' rather than always thinking that the living is going to happen somewhere beyond this embodiment, or thinking that as long as we have this embodiment we will be dying anyway?

Often when you ask questions, you ask it for this lifetime, which implicates that you believe that you only have this lifetime. What if you can ask for something now that can show up in different lifetimes, and you have no point of view about receiving it beyond this lifetime?

YOU CAN DIE MORE CONSCIOUS THAN MOST PEOPLE LIVE!

I'm so grateful to you for reading this. While I'm writing this, I can literally perceive the charge around this changing the Universe and, really, I am asking for full choice around death, life, living, and disease.
What do I mean by that – that you can have a full conscious choice?

This is the Body I'm going to have, this is the Body I'm going to leave, this is the moment I'm going to have it, this is the moment I'm going to leave it, this is what I will create in the meantime.

What this does is eliminate every need for disease, because the disease is always part of trying to fight you out of a no choice Universe, where you either must suffer, or you have decided you have no other possibility. For example, cancer, and I'm talking about the cancer that really kills people (not every cancer will eventually kill people, but most do because of the point of view that if they have the cancer, it will kill them). There are a few cancer forms that really break down the Body quite aggressively and very quickly. And what you see with that is people have decided that they want to die. They want to escape whatever they are in. There are people that die from cancer, because they want to die out of their marriage. Because they can't leave their partner or whatever they've decided. Death for them is an escape route, which will always be based on the point of view that you cannot make a different choice with ease.

YOU ALWAYS HAVE ANOTHER CHOICE!

Are you willing to commit to you, knowing that you have access to a completely different world than you are led and meant to believe? That every single molecule in the Universe desires to gift to you?

Are you willing to live as if you were just born and about to Die?

Are you willing to be out of control and beyond Judgment?

ARE YOU WILLING TO BE FREE?

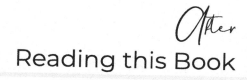

After Reading this Book

What I would suggest is getting this fancy magical process called "Access Bars" run.

I like to call it the Magic Touch that allows you to be greater and have way more ease than normal.

You can find more out about the Magic of Access Bars at
www.accessconsciousness.com/accessbars/

Also I would love for you to write a declaration of love to your Body!

Just imagine...This is your first day on this planet in this wonderful Body.

You just got it as a GIFT...

Let's open up to the space of really receiving this gift.

Unwrap it slowly...

Be amazed by the beauty of it...

Look at it...

Smell it...

Touch it...

Be with it...

What would you say to your beautiful Body?

Remember that you (even if you are unwilling to acknowledge it) picked this gift yourself. It is not something that someone else thought would be a great gift for you and you have no clue what to do with it.

Nope, it is a gift that you singlehandedly chose.

MY DECLARATION OF LOVE

Dear Body,

Have I ignored you...? Have I rejected you...? Have I abused you...? Have I diminished you...? Have I tried to kill you...?

Yes I have... all of the above and more...

Am I grateful that you did not kick me out...? Am I grateful for you being patient with my stupidity...? Am I amazed by your Magic and Capacities...? Am I grateful for you having my back showing me the true beauty of consciousness and living...?

Yes, I am... all of the above and more...

Here I am, right here right now, acknowledging your brilliance, your beauty, your power and your magic.

Body, you are amazing beyond words and although I might forget sometimes (or way too often), you are the gift that makes this life on this planet worth living.

You are a key to the everything that I never dared dreaming was possible.

You are a gift that keeps on giving.

I promise to more and more let go of all my judgments, all my lies, and all my projections that make you less instead of more...

I promise I keep reaching for communion rather than separation between us.

I promise to listen and allow you to override my annoying limited thoughts.

I promise to honor and trust you, to be vulnerable with you, and to ever cultivate gratitude for you.

I promise to be great today and greater tomorrow and every day from now on.

Dear Body, you are a gift that I will keep unwrapping as long as I choose to live with you!

Body, show me the way...

IT NEVER SHOWS UP THE WAY YOU THINK IT WILL!

About the *Author*

Together with co-facilitator puppy, Joy, Saskia Mevis is conquering the world. She loves to laugh, be MAGICAL, have fun with other crazy people, and enjoy life overall. She is the walking, talking SPACE that allows others to be everything they are.

Saskia is an Access Consciousness® Certified Facilitator specializing in Bodies and Awareness.

Her unique story and way of looking at the world will either inspire you or scare the bejesus out of you! ☺

Find out more:

   www.saskiamevis.com

May I Be a
Contribution to You?

Over the years I have trained and developed myself to work with my own unique capacities. I won't tell you what to do and I won't be able to fix you! What I will do is empower you to know what will create the change that you desire to create. If I am the energy that you are looking for, I would love to get together and see what we can change.

CONSCIOUSNESS GIFTS YOU POSSIBILITIES WHEN THIS REALITY SAYS THERE ARE NONE...

What does Consciousness mean to me?
Consciousness, for me, is the space in the world, where there is no right or wrong and people can actually be free from all

the trauma, drama, and suffering. A space where there is a possibility for everyone to live with Ease, Joy, and Glory and to change everything that doesn't work for them.

EVERY MOVE YOU MAKE MOVES EVERYTHING!
Everything is connected!
We consist out of trillions of molecules, each of which in turn is individually connected to the quantum field. This is your entrance to the universal law of Infinite Possibilities. Every molecule in the universe is connected to everything in a great space of infinity, far beyond what you can understand with your mind. Your thoughts, intentions and movements not only move you, but also everything around you.

How much vulnerability, power, gratitude and joy can you move in the world to be the greatest contribution to yourself, your Body, your life and the Earth?

In that movement, where there are no judgments, definitions, and expectations, is the infinite space of possibilities that you and your Body truly are. Who you are and the possibilities you have, have not existed on this planet before.

If this is for you, and you are ready to take the leap, check out the infinite possibilities:

 www.saskiamevis.com/choosetolive

YOUR BODY IS WILLING TO HAVE YOUR BACK;
ARE YOU WILLING TO HAVE YOURS?

Additional *Resources*

WHAT WILL IT TAKE FOR YOU TO SEE WHAT UNIQUE GIFT YOU TRULY ARE AND CHANGE THE WORLD BY BEING EXACTLY THAT?

I found a YouTube video that I recorded 6 months after the diagnosis. I cannot even put into words how much everything has changed, and what a GIFT the past years have been to me!

Beautiful You...in case you need a reminder today...

CONSCIOUSNESS MAKES EVERYTHING GREATER, ALWAYS!

 How my life changed from one day on to another... disaster or gift?

Made in the USA
Las Vegas, NV
01 May 2023

71415653R00063